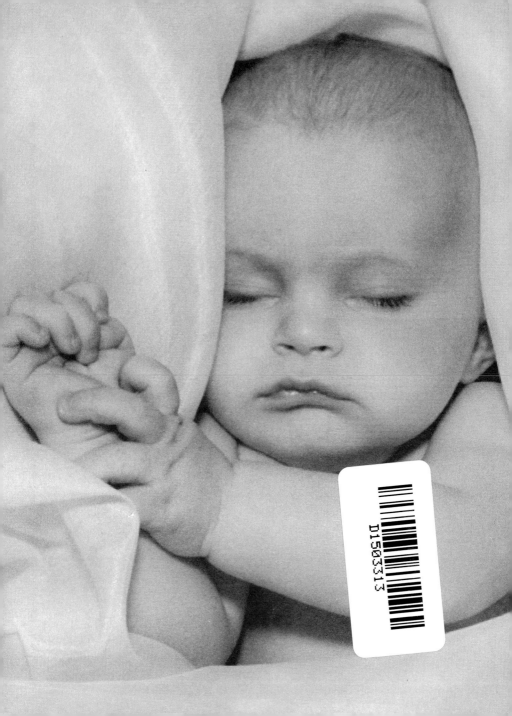

52
SLEEP SECRETS FOR BABIES

52

SLEEP SECRETS
FOR BABIES

KIM WEST

The Sleep Lady®

Author of *Good Night, Sleep Tight*

With love and gratitude to Carleigh and Gretchen,
my precious daughters and my first priceless teachers
of these sleep secrets; to the thousands of families,
who have laughed, cried and celebrated their struggles
and progress with me over the years and unknowingly
helped me build the foundation for this book.

Contents

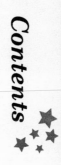

Foreword

by Dr. Lisa Thebner

At a newborn's first doctor's visit, parents are filled with joy, wonderment, pride, and, of course, trepidation about caring for their little baby. Among the many issues facing new parents are questions about feeding, diapering, bathing, and soothing techniques.

A major question on most parents' minds is when and how their baby is going to sleep. As a pediatrician, I spend a significant amount of time talking about sleep with my families. Such things as how much their baby should be sleeping, how to get their baby to go to sleep, and how to break bad sleeping habits are the most common themes.

I first heard about the Sleep Lady® from a family in my practice. Worn out from sleepless nights and preferring to avoid the "cry it out" approach to sleep training, these parents had actively sought out and found another method of coaxing their little one into naps during the day and sleeping well at night. Their alternative technique was one developed by Kim West, the Sleep Lady®, who helped them turn their baby into a well-rested, easy-to-put-down baby. In regard to sleep training, their lives, as well as my own practice, have not been the same since. "She gave us our lives back!" and "She changed our lives!" are direct quotes from ecstatic (and well-rested) parents who have worked with Kim.

I start talking early on with families about the importance of sleep. Proper sleep is crucial for an overall healthy child—not to mention healthy parents! Our first conversation often happens during a prenatal visit. Like many problems in medicine, prevention can be an important key to success. I stress the importance of valuing sleep and developing a routine that prepares the parents for what they may expect as their baby grows. I recommend certain books, including *Good Night, Sleep Tight*, by Kim West.

Now, Kim's new, easy-to-use book becomes another helpful tool for helping your baby to "sleep like a baby." *52 Sleep Secrets for Babies* is a comprehensive and succinct guide to so many of the issues that pediatricians would love to cover extensively in the office if they had the time, issues that parents want to hear about. I will be enthusiastically recommending this excellent book to my new parents.

I've seen countless families who have benefited from the principles outlined in this book. Now you and your baby will, too. You are on your way to a sleep-filled night and a happier day!

Introduction

"I had no idea that sleep could be so elusive!"

"I thought my baby would just magically sleep through the night."

"If I'd known how important it was to teach my kids to sleep, I would have done things differently."

I'm Kim West, also known as the Sleep Lady®, and I've written *52 Sleep Secrets for Babies* for the many, many new parents who find themselves thinking exactly these things, and more, when it comes to their children and sleep. After all, sleep is everything—that is, when you're not getting enough it sure feels like that! Call me biased, but I find that if baby *and* parents are sleeping well everyone is a *lot* happier! A well-rested baby is usually an easier, less cranky baby. A well-rested mom or dad is an easier, less cranky parent—able to keep frustration and irritation at bay and be more loving and joyful.

I'm the mother of two girls, and have been a family therapist for fifteen years. Through my personal life and my work, I have been blessed with hands-on experience with all kinds of parenting and sleep issues, and from those experiences I've distilled many secrets to help make the first few years of parenting a bit easier. Neither of my daughters was an "angel baby" who just drifted off each night into peaceful slumber. Still, I had the oldest, Carleigh, sleeping through the night (by that I mean for eight-hour stretches) at eight weeks. Gretchen, my youngest, was sleeping through the night by ten weeks—even though she posed some special challenges: she was fussy and had reflux. And yes, I breast-fed both of them. I started helping friends teach their babies and toddlers to sleep, and then helped friends of friends. Word spread, and soon I had a growing number of sleepy parents with sleepless babies knocking on my door. My private practice began to focus more and more on such families.

As a result, my Sleep Lady approach is founded on my general beliefs as a family therapist: I'm a proponent of developing and maintaining a secure attachment with a child while creating a family life where *everyone* is happy, healthy and well rested. My sleep approach builds on step-by-step changes in bedtime, napping and overnight routines so that a child can develop sleep independence and sleep more soundly and longer, feeling confident that Mom and Dad will be nearby and responsive. It's a gentler alternative for families who can't stomach the idea of letting their babies cry it out; for families who have tried Ferber without success; and for families who had success earlier with crying it out but find that it isn't working now. I have also worked with families who believe in co-sleeping but whose babies don't really sleep all that well nestled snugly with Mom and Dad. And I've guided many families who did co-sleep for a few months or a few years but now want the family bed to revert to a marital one.

52 Sleep Secrets for Babies summarizes much of what I have learned from working with thousands of families and now teach to new parents I see in my practice and meet through my website. So many parents have asked me for a quick and easy-to-follow guide to help their babies learn to sleep and help them prevent problems down the road that I have put together this little book. You can carry it with you anywhere and refer to it before and after sleep problems arise.

I hope you find these golden sleep nuggets to be priceless!

Sweet dreams,
Kim West, LCSW-C
The Sleep Lady®

P.S. This book, actually, no book, is a substitute for seeing a pediatrician. You need to rule out any medical conditions that hamper sleep. Talk to your pediatrician about your baby's sleep problems and feeding patterns, and be sure to mention any digestive difficulties, allergies, noisy breathing, or snoring. And if you're looking for a full blown, step-by-step gentle method for sleep coaching your child, take a look at **Good Night, Sleep Tight: The Sleep Lady's Gentle Guide to Helping Your Child Go to Sleep, Stay Asleep, and Wake Up Happy**

Visit my website, www.sleeplady.com, for ongoing news and more tips on sleep and parenting, as well as for announcements of upcoming 52 Sleep Secrets books on toddlers, school-age children and adult sleep!

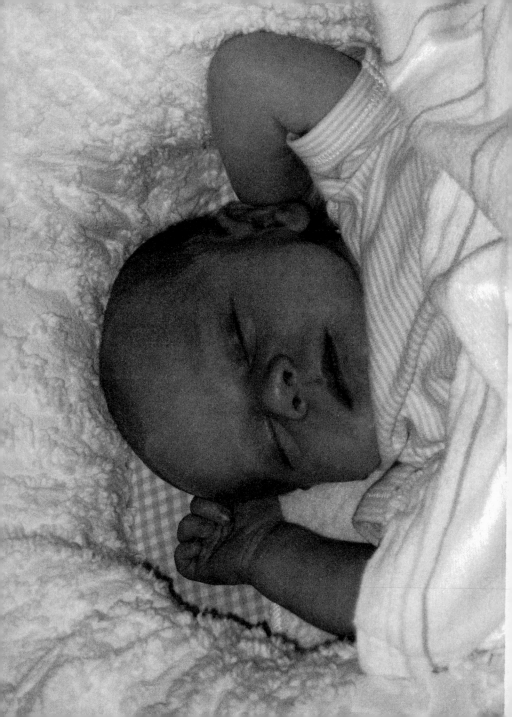

General Secrets

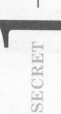

SECRET

1

Getting enough sleep will help baby grow, learn, and stay well.

Sleep is vital to health and development. While your baby sleeps, her body is

- Producing growth hormones

- Building up her immune system

- Retaining, storing and organizing memories—the building blocks of learning.

2

2

Babies need A LOT of sleep!

Here's how much snooze time a baby should log over 24 hours meaning at night and at nap time as he grows:

1 week	16.5 hours
1 month	15.5 hours
3 months	15 hours
6 months	14.25 hours
9 months	14 hours
12 months	13.75 hours
18 months	13.5 hours

SECRET 3

Alert, bright babies need MORE than the average amount of sleep—not less.

A baby who seems ahead of the curve—interested in the world around her, reaching milestones early—often fools her parents into thinking she needs less sleep than the "typical" baby. In fact, she needs more. Because she's so engaged with her surroundings, she often has a harder time shutting down. She's "too busy" to bother going to sleep...or so it seems! This kind of baby also knows what she wants and when she wants it, and she's willing to hold out until she gets it. She can be a little tough to parent. She especially needs you to make sure she gets the sleep she needs but won't admit to needing. Since this type of baby is often able to hide her sleepy cues, you must watch the clock and get her into bed on time. And keep in mind that she probably won't be a flexible sleeper for several years, meaning she'll need utter consistency when it comes to when, where and how she goes to sleep.

4

4

It takes an average of 15 to 20 minutes to fall asleep.

This applies to grown-ups and babies alike. Experts say that if you're "asleep before your head hits the pillow," you're probably sleep-deprived. So keep this in mind if you think your baby is taking too long to settle down, and don't rush to "rescue" him. It may take him 15 or 20 minutes to land in La-La Land.

5

Babies do all sorts of things to soothe themselves to sleep.

Some typical rituals:

- Sucking on thumbs, fingers, a pacifier, or a lovey
  - Twirling the tags or ears of stuffed toys
    - Twirling their own hair
- Playing with their ears (not just a sign of ear infections)
  - Rubbing their blanket or lovey against their face
    - Rocking their body or head
- Gently banging their head, legs or arms against the crib bumper
  - Lifting their legs up and letting them drop
    - Humming, singing, babbling or talking
      - Weaving their blankie between their fingers

6

Babies are notoriously "light" sleepers.

Just like grown-ups and older kids, infants switch between REM (light) sleep and non-REM (very deep) sleep several times during the night and during naps. The difference is, until they're around two years old, babies log more REM sleep, which is when they dream, and also when they may wake up a bit. It's during such partial arousals they may realize they can't get back to sleep—unless, that is, they've learned how. That's why it's important for a baby to be able to put herself to sleep—otherwise she'll need you to come help her every time she wakes up.

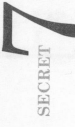

7

Babies need both quality and quantity of sleep.

This means getting:

- The right kind of sleep—unfragmented, uninterrupted and "motionless." Don't wake your baby to eat unless he physically needs to eat, and no rocking, swinging or car riding, as movement keeps the brain in a lighter sleep, which is not as restorative to the brain as a deep sleep.

- The right timing—as in consistent bedtimes, wake-up times and nap times.

- The right amount of sleep (see Secret #2 for the average sleep requirements for kids of different ages). Your child shouldn't vary from these numbers by more than an hour.

8

Nobody puts you to sleep at night, so your baby needs to learn to do it, too.

You figured out a long time ago the tricks that help you fall asleep: a warm bath, a good book, imagining something pleasant—like walking along a beautiful beach. Your baby will also need to learn how to drift off by herself.

Teaching her how is your job.

9

Sleep develops in a specific order.

This means you'll start seeing a glimmer of a sleep schedule, starting with:

1. Night sleep—at around 6 to 8 weeks in a healthy full-term newborn

2. Morning nap—at around 12 weeks

3. Afternoon nap—at around 16 weeks

10

When it comes to where, when and how their baby sleeps moms and dads need to be on the same page.

You can't cleanly separate sleep from other areas of parenting. If you make a plan and then can't follow through together, it's unfair to your child. For instance, if Mom wants the baby to sleep in the family bed, and Dad wants the baby to sleep in her crib, it's just not going to work. Think it through. Talk it through. Discuss how much crying each of you can tolerate, and what your parenting styles are. Find goals and approaches you can agree on, and then share them with any caregivers who'll be spending a lot of time with your baby.

SECRET 11

Make sleep a family priority.

In our society, it's not hard to fill up an entire day with one errand or obligation after another. Naps and reasonable bedtimes usually get short shrift—and not just for your baby. When it's clear that the whole family's not logging enough zzzz's, it's time to make sleep a priority. Work your schedule around your baby's (and older children's) nap times, even if it means telling friends and relatives that you're not available to visit or get together (for now). Just tell them you need your sleep—they'll understand...

And try to get everyone home in the evenings in plenty of time for dinner, bedtime routines and lights out. After all, happy, well-rested children make for happy, well-rested parents.

12

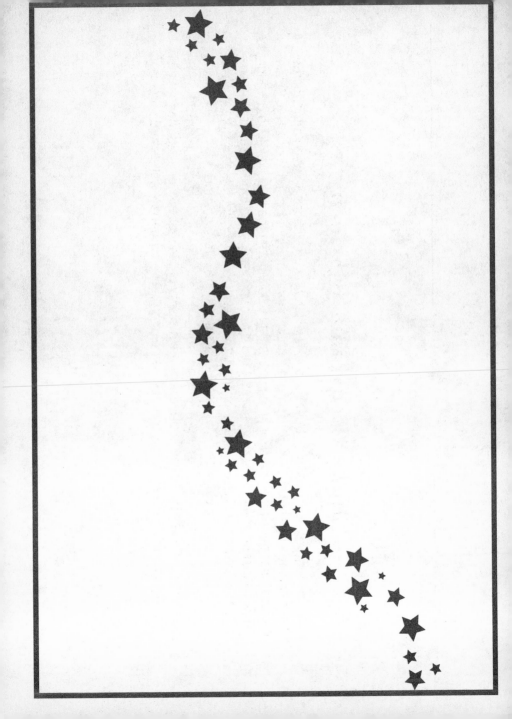

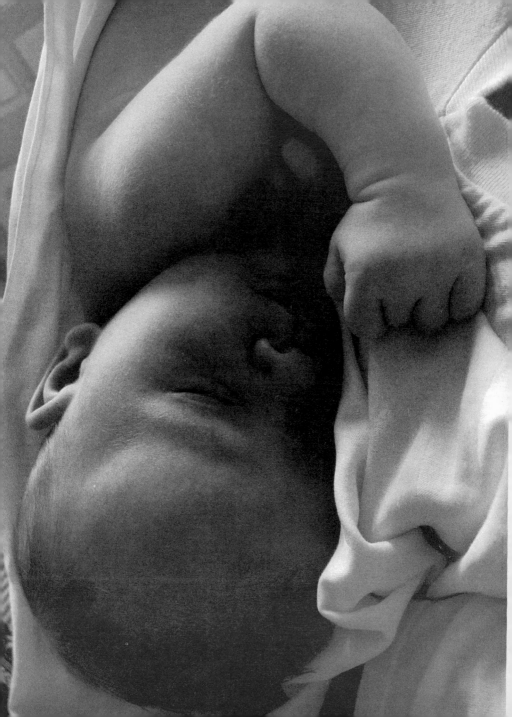

Setting The Stage For Good Sleep Habits

SECRET

12

Your baby will rest best in a "sleep-friendly" room.

It's fun to decorate a nursery: the sweet bedding! adorable toys! lovely shower gifts! Go ahead and make your baby's room as cute as can be, but be sure to incorporate a few elements that will help guarantee he'll be able to sleep in it:

- Walls painted soft, neutral or pale colors

- A dimmer on the overhead light or lamp—so you won't have to perform those wee hour feedings and diaper changes under glaring lights

    - A night-light

    - Room-darkening shades

- Thermostat set between 68 and 72 degrees Fahrenheit

- A white-noise machine, especially if you have older children, a dog that barks a lot or if you live in a noisy neighborhood

    - A crib with a firm mattress

- Keep stimulating toys, like black-and-white mobiles, out of the crib

16

13

Your baby needs a soothing bedtime routine.

This will tell her that it's time to slow down. The ideal pre-sleep ritual for a baby lasts no more than 20 to 30 minutes—otherwise you'll be asleep before it's over! It may include two or three activities, such as:

- A warm bath
- Infant massage (in the baby's room, with the lights low)
- Playing soft music or singing her a lullaby
- A snack (nursing or a bottle)
- Burping
- Swaddling
- A snuggle and kisses

You can add books when your baby is around six months old. Whatever you do, do it in the same order each night. Babies find predictability comforting. And a comfy baby is a happy sleeper.

14

There's no reason for your baby to "get used to" sleeping with bright lights on or loud noises in the background.

You may have been told by well-intended family, friends or strangers to condition your baby to sleep with lights glaring and vacuum blaring. Don't listen! Can you fall asleep with a lot of noise in the background? We all sleep better in the dark and in the quiet—and in a comfortable bed (see Secret #12). A dim night-light is okay (under 7 watts) so you can easily check on your baby.

If you're worried that your baby will become "addicted" to the sound of a noise machine, turn it off when you go to bed, or slowly reduce the volume. Most children start sleeping more deeply by age two, so you may find that your preschooler sleeps just fine surrounded by noise.

18

15

A video monitor can save you trips to the nursery.

Once your baby is sleeping in her own room—whether right from the start or after she's outgrown the bassinet or co-sleeper in your room—you may find yourself rushing to check on her every time she stirs. Or you may just plain worry because you can't see her. Here's where a video monitor comes in handy. You'll be able to see when she really needs you, and just as important, when she really doesn't. You'll sleep better, and she'll have more opportunities to perfect her self-soothing skills.

16

A TV in the nursery or bedroom disturbs the peace.

Television is the number-one sleep crutch for adults in this country. Watching the tube puts the brain into a light trance, similar to the first stages of sleep. Grown-ups who rely on the TV to help them fall asleep will often have to turn it back on if they wake up during the night and can't drop off again. Given that experts recommend reducing kids' tube time in general, do you really want your child to become dependent on TV at bedtime? And don't forget that as children get older they learn to switch on the television by themselves— if there's a TV in their bedroom, you won't be able to monitor what they see and when.

SECRET

17

It's best to shed a little light on the pre-sleep routine.

Don't nurse or give your baby her bottle in complete darkness. She's more likely to fall asleep before she's filled up her tummy—and you won't be able to see her if she does.

Remember: Drowsy but awake!

Turn on a night-light, lamp or an overhead light that can be dimmed.

18

A baby who co-sleeps with mom and dad should still log some snooze time in his own bed.

Put your baby in his crib or bassinette for at least one nap a day, especially if you plan to have him sleep there all the time after he's three to six months old (if you go back to work during this time, for example). This way he'll get acclimated to his room and bed, and he'll have a chance to learn to put himself to sleep independently.

You'll want to sleep when the baby sleeps during the first several weeks, but after a while you'll want to be able to get some things done during nap time.

22

19

Well-rested parents mean well-rested babies and kids.

Sleep deprivation can leave us irritable, impatient, sad, moody and forgetful—none of which is conducive to being the parent or partner we want to be. But when we get enough sleep (for the mom and dad of a newborn, that means a five-hour stretch), we have the energy and patience to do our job well—and that includes teaching our babies good sleep habits. You need to work as a team so that one of you can get those essential hours of zzzz's, especially if Mom is breast-feeding. Once the baby has been introduced to a bottle, Dad should take over one feeding per night at least several nights a week. The parent who's "off duty" may want to wear earplugs or sleep in a room that's away from the baby or baby monitor.

20

Massage is a wonderful sleep-inducer.

Babies need to be touched just as much as they need to be fed. When you hold and cuddle your baby, you're showing her you love her. And when you gently stroke and rub your baby, you help her to relax—just as a soothing massage relaxes you. Take an infant massage class at your hospital or birthing center, and be sure to bring Dad along—since he can't breast-feed, massage is a lovely and nurturing way for him to bond with the baby.

21

Certain sounds are conducive to sleep.

Researchers have identified some specific sounds that babies find especially comforting—and a relaxed baby is a baby who's able to drift off. Some things that are music to a newborn's ears:

- Mom's voice—talking soothingly or singing, even off-key

- The thumping of a heartbeat, which he listened to constantly before birth

  - The ocean

- Any tune with 60 or less beats per minute—they aren't called lull-abies for nothing!

22

Happy mommies and daddies raise happy babies—babies who sleep well at night.

One of the best gifts you can give your children is your own well-being. That includes making sure your own sleep habits are healthy:

- Get a little exercise each day—this will increase your happy hormones.
- Cut down on caffeine and alcohol. Drink a cup of chamomile tea to relax.
- Take a warm bath before bedtime. Lavender-scented bath salts will relax you even more.
  - Take naps (of 45- to 90-minutes) when you can.
  - Make sure your mattress is firm and comfortable.
  - Keep the thermostat between 68 and 72 degrees.
- Turn off the TV or computer, if you have either or both in your bedroom.
  - Get to bed early enough to be well rested in the morning.
- Before turning in, listen to quiet music, read a book, snuggle with your spouse.

Once you and your baby are starting to get a little bit more sleep, hire a sitter and get out of the house with your spouse—alone!

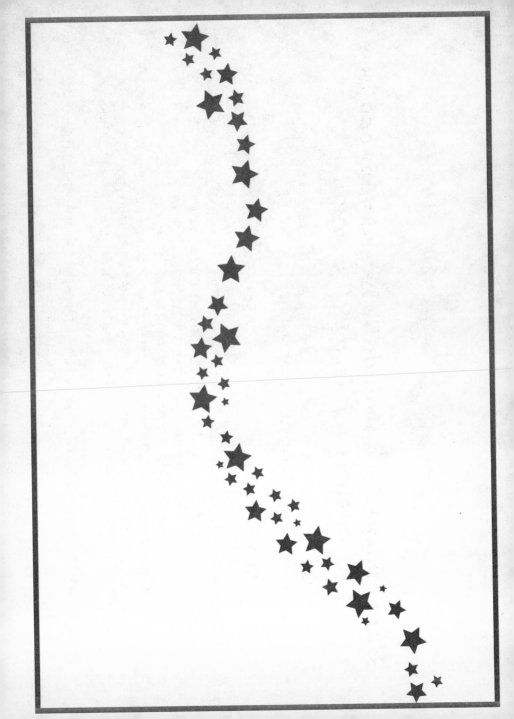

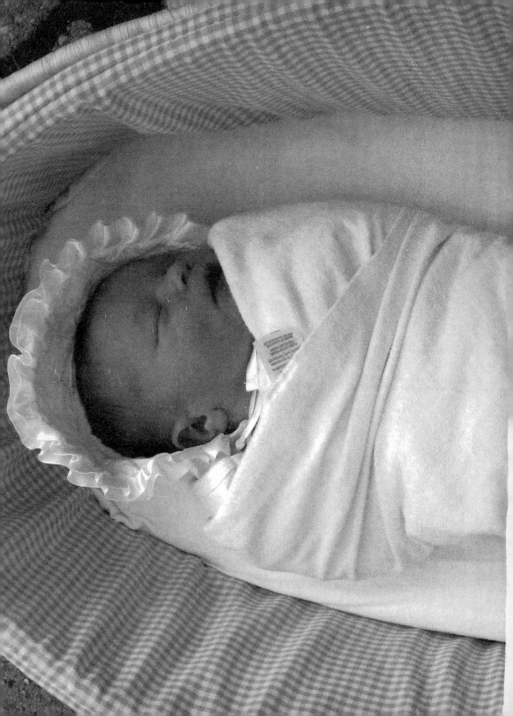

Specific to Newborns

23

You can start teaching your baby to sleep when he's two weeks old.

Really, you can! The first couple of weeks after your baby is born his sleep will be disorganized neurologically—which means it'll mostly be a light slumber. Trying to teach him to go to sleep by himself will be pointless. And besides, you'll have enough to do: letting your body heal, learning the basics like breast-feeding, diapering, swaddling. So when it comes to sleep, just do what feels right: hold him, rock him, sway with him. But around two weeks, you can start gradually laying the groundwork for the healthy sleep habits that your child can use for the rest of his life.

24

Newborns don't know night from day.

You'll have to help your baby learn the difference.

During the day …

- Keep the curtains open and the lights on when he's awake.
- Get outside when the weather's nice—research has found that exposure to sunlight during the day helps babies sleep better at night.
- Feed him every three hours—even if you have to wake him up.

During the night …

- Pull down the shades, dim the lights.
- Switch to quiet activities, like massage, quiet talking or singing, reading him a singsong book.
- Keep nighttime feedings brief and boring.

25

Sometimes it's okay to wake a sleeping baby.

During the day, that is. She shouldn't go longer than three hours without a meal, so wake her up if you must in order to avoid letting her get too hungry. Save those long stretches of sleep for nighttime—and enjoy them!

26

Your baby's body knows best when it needs to sleep.

Just like adults and older kids, your baby has an internal clock that dictates when she should be awake and when her body needs to sleep. If she skips a necessary siesta (during the day or during the night), her body will secrete a hormone called cortisol, which acts like a mild form of adrenaline. She'll become too wound up to sleep—even if you put her to bed. She'll cry more than usual, take longer to finally doze off, and sleep fitfully; what's more, under the influence of the cortisol coursing through her body, she'll wake up more often during the night and earlier the next morning. It doesn't take many missed sleep periods before she's in a downward spiral—physically unable to sleep when she needs to, prompting the release of more cortisol, and so on. Watch for cues that your baby is sleepy. Watch the clock, too. Newborns need to sleep every one and a half to two hours.

27

Maybe he can't talk yet, but your baby can signal when he's sleepy.

Watch for these signs that it's nap or bedtime:

- Eye-rubbing
- Yawning
- "Slowing down" during play
- Fussiness, even when he's been fed
- Thumb-sucking (if he's a thumb-sucker)
- Caressing his lovey or security object
- Asking for a pacifier, a bottle or to nurse even if he has recently been fed
- A glazed look in his eyes

28

A flexible routine is better than a rigid schedule.

Here's how it goes: Every baby is different, and every parent feels differently about keeping a schedule. For some moms, a time for everything and everything in its time is key to making it through the day. For others, figuring out a schedule is too much work—and adhering to one is sheer torture! They also may not feel right about "imposing" a schedule on their babies. That said, all babies like predictability; it's comforting for them to know what's coming next. And even if you don't like schedules, you can come up with a routine that's flexible. In fact, it will help you figure out the best times to schedule appointments, make plans with friends, do the grocery shopping.

To develop a flexible routine: Keep a log of how often your baby eats and when. Watch to see when your child's sleep windows naturally occur, so that you can plan around when she needs to nap.

With a routine in place, you will be better able to "read" your baby when she cries: if you know by her built-in schedule when she's usually hungry or sleepy, you'll know what all the wailing means and be able to act on it promptly. That will be a relief to both of you.

35

29

Babies don't only cry when they're hungry.

They cry when they're uncomfortable, bored, overstimulated, and yes, when they're sleepy. So unless it's a time when she usually eats, don't automatically offer your baby a breast or bottle the second she starts to whimper. Check her diaper, give her a change of scenery. If you suspect she missed her last opportunity to nap and now she's too riled to settle down, try these calming techniques:

- Take her into a quiet room and dim the lights.
  - Swaddle her.
- Hold her in a football hold (snuggled against your side), and sway with her.
  - Make shushing noises.
  - Offer her a pacifier.

If she cries a lot and you can't figure out what's wrong, check with your pediatrician to make sure she doesn't have an underlying medical condition, such as reflux, that might be causing her discomfort.

SECRET

30

You can't spoil a baby by going to him when he cries.

Indeed, if you don't respond to your baby, he may get the message he's not important. Taking care of his needs isn't the same as coddling. It's vital to developing a secure attachment—in other words, he'll know that when he cries someone always comes. And a secure attachment is key to healthy self-esteem later in life.

So when your baby cries, give him a few seconds to settle down, then check to see what might be bothering him:

- Is he hungry? How long has it been since he last ate?

- Is his diaper wet or poopy?

- Is he too hot or too cold?

- Is he sick?

- Is he overstimulated?

- Is he overtired? Has he been awake more than two hours?

31

A baby who can roll over will be a more independent sleeper.

Since babies sleep on their backs, they don't get much chance to exercise the muscles in their necks and upper bodies that they'll need to roll over, sit up, crawl, and walk. So when your baby is awake, put him on his tummy (in a safe place, like on a blanket on the floor) for a few minutes every day. He'll naturally lift his head to take a look around. As he gets older, you can hold a mirror or toy just out of reach to encourage him. The sleep advantage is this: As your baby gets stronger, he will be better able to reposition himself to get more comfortable in the night. Eventually he will be able to roll over, and even reach for his lovey or pacifier.

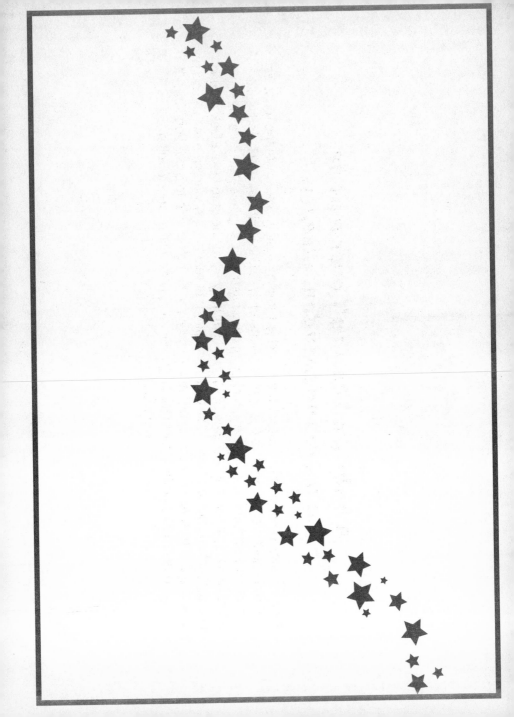

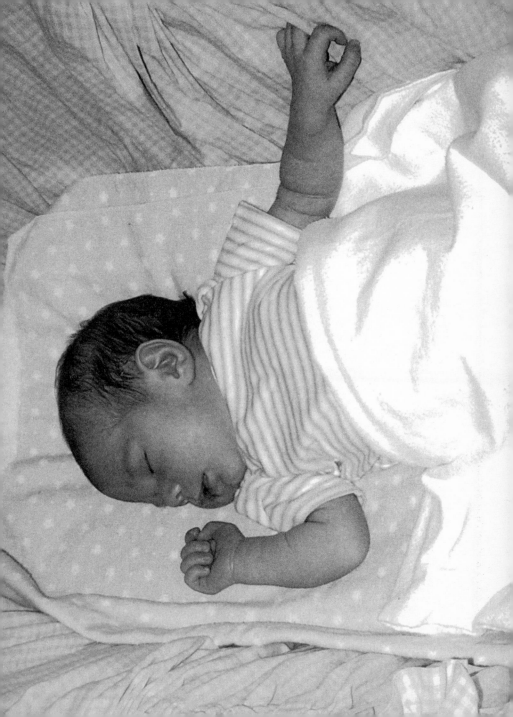

Specific to Babies
4 to 8 Weeks and Older

32

Buckle your seat belt when your baby is about a month old: you may be in for a bumpy ride.

At about four weeks, many babies enter a super-fussy period that peaks at around six weeks and wanes by about twelve weeks. This is because at this age babies are too old to shut out stimulation (or habituate)—that is, they're too aware of what's going on around them. At the same time, they haven't yet mastered any self-calming techniques. This is the period when colic can set in, too—and the result is crying and fussiness, usually in the late afternoon and early evening. It's not the best time for visitors or outings, so plan accordingly. Stay home, alone, turn down the lights, and let your baby have a late-afternoon snooze. You'll both feel better!

33

Mealtimes and bedtimes don't always mix.

Which is to say, you don't want your baby to rely on the breast or bottle every single time she goes to sleep. As often as you can during the day, feed her when she wakes up—not as part of her nap-time routine. In the evening, when she's getting that last meal before a nice long stretch of sleep, do what you can to keep her awake until her tummy's full. If those baby blues start to flutter closed and her sucking gets weaker, talk to her gently, or rub her palms or the bottoms of her feet to rouse her. When she finishes eating, burp her, kiss her, and put her to bed. If you can't keep her awake during that last feeding, try doing it earlier—perhaps before her bath.

34

You can put your baby to bed drowsy but awake when he is six to eight weeks old.

Because his nighttime sleep is becoming more organized (meaning it's going through distinct REM and non-REM cycles), this is the perfect time for your baby to begin to learn the last part of falling asleep on his own. If you put him down when he's completely asleep, he will miss this learning opportunity.

35

"Drowsy but awake" means your baby is aware she's being put down.

Besides relaxed and sleepy, the "drowsy" part means your baby feels loved, cozy and warm, has a dry diaper and a full tummy, and her room is dim. The "awake" part means she knows that you're putting her down in her crib, bassinet, or co-sleeper. She may squirm and fuss a bit before she falls asleep—that's okay. You can stay nearby, talk to her and rub her back intermittently until she's out.

36

Don't put your baby down TOO drowsy.

If your baby goes right to sleep at nap and bedtime but wakes frequently and/or shortly after he goes to bed, then he may be too sleepy when you put him down. In other words, he looks like he's still awake, but really, he's so far gone that when his head hits the crib he conks right out and doesn't actually spend any time actively putting himself to sleep. You'll have to fine-tune your understanding of his body language to figure out exactly when it's best to put him down. Start by putting him down when he's obviously more awake than usual. He might fuss—remember, he's not really used to this! Stay with him, talk to him. You can shush him, tell him it's okay, it's time to go night-night, sing a gentle song and pat or rub his back. Do this intermittently until he falls asleep. Then apply this process to nap times.

37

If your baby gets hooked on a sleep "crutch," eventually bedtime will be your nightmare.

It's fine to rock, walk, feed, sing to or pat your baby to help her settle down before sleep, or to reassure her if she's having trouble drifting off by herself. But after she is six to eight weeks old, don't do these things until she conks out. She'll learn that the only way she can fall asleep is if you are doing them. That goes double for when she wakes up in the middle of the night. Once she's relaxed and calm, put her in her crib while she's still awake and let her finish the trip to Dreamland by herself.

38

A wee-hour feeding is not an invitation to party.

When you feed your baby in the middle of the night, don't make it fun. Keep the lights off or low, don't play with her, don't even change her diaper unless she's poopy.

If she tends to get really soaked during the night, consider using a larger-size diaper with an "insert" or "doubler"—a pad you can add to the diaper to bump up its absorbency. These are great for long car or plane trips as well, by the way.

Just feed her, burp her, kiss her, and then put her right back into her bed—not yours!

48

39

"Motion sleep" is not the best sleep.

Sure, your baby conks out in the car or stroller or swing. And for the first six to eight weeks, that's okay. But after that, snoozing-on-the-go all the time is a no-no: motion lulls babies to sleep, but it keeps them in a light, fragmented sleep—not the restorative cyclic sleep during which the brain stores memories and the immune system gets a boost. If your baby does fall asleep while riding in the car or stroller, transfer him to his crib as soon as you can.

Or, you could just park the car in your driveway and flip through a magazine or pay bills while he snoozes.

SECRET 40

Dads are excellent at bedtime routines.

Take turns with your partner putting your baby to bed. If nursing isn't an element of her bedtime routine, this will be easy. Even if you're breast-feeding, though, there's no reason to ban Dad from the nursery. After you nurse, hand him the baby for burping, swaddling, and the rest of the nightly ritual. He'll probably come up with his own versions of soothing techniques—and that's just fine!

And while Dad finishes up with the baby, you can spend quality time with your older kids, if you have them, or just put your feet up and relax. You deserve it!

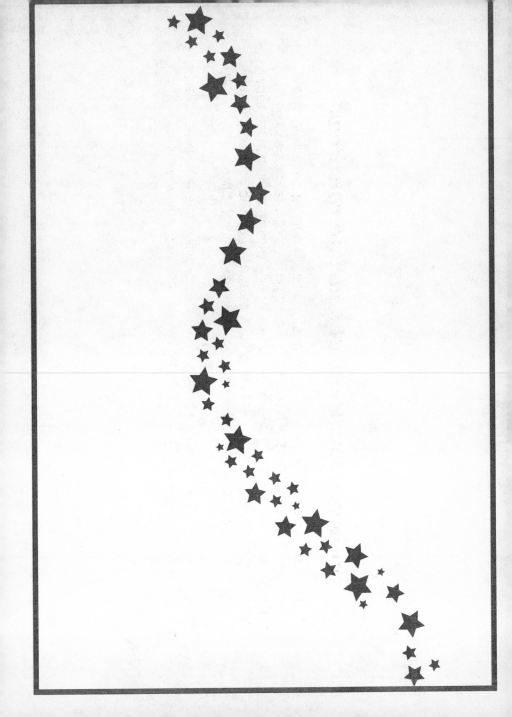

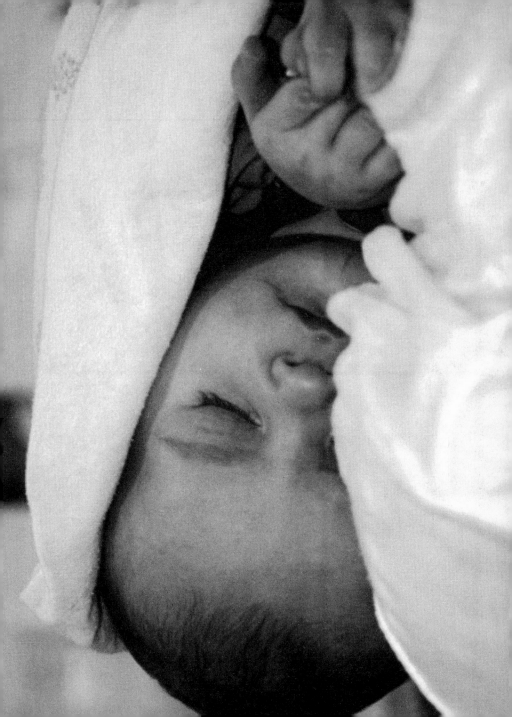

Specific to Babies
12 Weeks and Older

41

A daytime schedule starts to appear around three months.

Your baby will begin producing melatonin, a hormone that regulates the body's internal clock, at around three months. Finally, you'll start to see a glimmer of regularity in the times he sleeps, eats, and is alert. You may notice that he's consistently ready to sleep around 8 or 9 p.m., whereas up until now his bedtime was all over the place. Then you'll notice that he takes his morning nap around 9 a.m., or about one and a half to two hours after he wakes up. Now you can put together a flexible schedule.

42

Naps are better taken at home.

At three to four months, your baby is becoming more alert and aware of her surroundings. Napping "on the go" doesn't work very well anymore. She needs a quiet, dimly lit environment in which to shut down and go to sleep—specifically, her own crib in her own room.

Plan outings and errands around nap time, or hire a sitter to stay with your sleeping baby if you must be out during her usual siestas.

43

Less daytime sleep means less nighttime sleep.

It's not a typo—but it is a conundrum. You can't get a baby to sleep more at night by keeping her up during the day. It's that pesky cortisol again. Remember: If your baby doesn't get to nap when she needs to, her body produces cortisol, which revs her up and makes sleeping even harder and less restful.

44

Babies sleep better if they sleep with a "friend."

By "friend" I mean a security object, or "lovey." It could be a stuffed animal, a favorite blanket, or even a cloth diaper or one of your T-shirts. It will help your baby feel safe and secure if she has her lovey when you're not around—for example, when she wakes in the middle of the night. If by the time she's six months old your baby hasn't fallen in love with something on her own, encourage her as part of sleep coaching. Choose something cuddly and soft; make sure it's small but not so small she could choke on it, and not so large that she could use it to climb out of her crib or get stuck underneath it. Let her hold it while she nurses; play peek-a-boo with it at playtime. Make it come alive for your baby. If she rejects your first choice, try with something else. Eventually you'll hit on that special something. Consider buying duplicates, if possible; loveys are notorious for going astray at shopping malls.

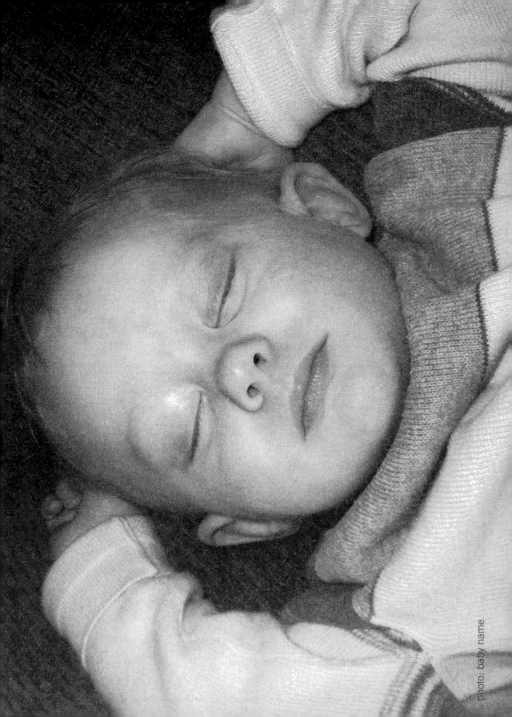

Specific to Toddlers
"Thinking Ahead"

45

On average, toddlers who are sleeping through the night switch from two naps to one between 15 and 18 months.

Signs your child may be ready for this change:

- He's been consistently sleeping through the night (11 solid hours) for at least three weeks.
  - It's taking longer and longer for him to fall asleep at morning nap time.
- His morning naps are getting shorter and shorter (or longer, but he refuses to take an afternoon nap).

If you think your child is ready to drop his morning nap, then start pushing it later and later, by 15 to 30 minutes, to 12:30 or 1 p.m., over seven to ten days. He'll need an earlier bedtime (between 7 and 7:30 is ideal) during this transition.

46

The best time to graduate a toddler from crib to big-kid bed is at two and a half to three years old.

Before then, your child won't understand what "stay in your bed all night long" means: she may decide to get up and wander around the house in the middle of the night. Not only that, making the switch too soon usually exacerbates existing sleep problems if there are any. If, however, you're going to need the crib for a new baby before your older child is two and a half, make the transition at least two months before or four months after the new sibling arrives, so big sib won't feel as if she's being kicked out of her crib and replaced.

Better yet, if your toddler or preschooler isn't ready to give up the crib, don't push it. Borrow one for the new baby, or buy one secondhand.

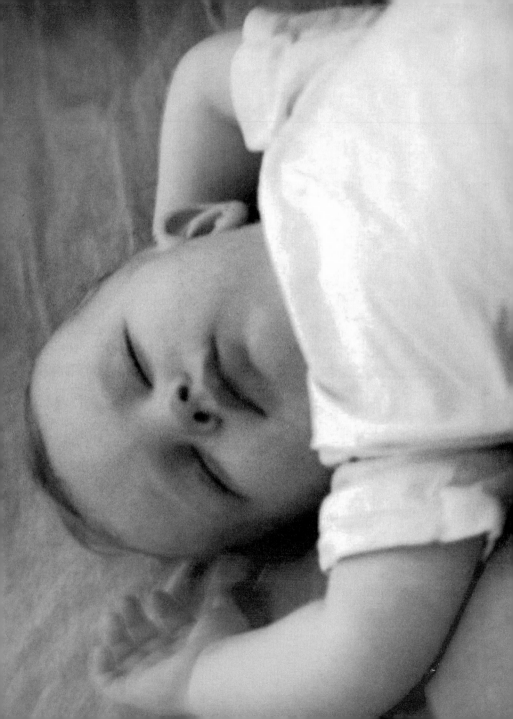

General Sleep Coaching Tips

47

The right training method is essential for sleep success.

Research suggests that the most effective method of sleep training is "extinction"—in other words, putting a baby in his crib awake, then leaving the room and letting him cry himself to sleep, no matter how long it takes. Well, it does work—because if you really stick to your guns and don't respond at all to your baby, you don't risk responding inconsistently. The message here: You need to find a sleep-coaching approach that is the right match for your baby's or child's temperament and your own tolerance for tears, and then follow through patiently and consistently.

48

Pick the ideal time to start sleep coaching.

If your baby is six months or older and you didn't gently "shape" her sleep from the beginning, it's not too late to start now. Time it wisely, though: It will take about three weeks to teach her to put herself to sleep. Avoid times when there are potential disruptions—like teething, travel or moving. Many parents like to start on a Friday night. That way, if one or both work, they'll both be around on the weekend for the first few days of coaching.

Whichever night you choose as Night Number One, do your best to make sure your baby gets in enough nap time during the day.

49

Keeping a feeding-and-sleep log is key to sleep coaching.

Here's what you should keep track of:

- What time you put your baby to bed
- How long it takes him to get to sleep

- How long he cries before finally conking out. Remember, five minutes of crying can feel like 50, which is why it's helpful to time it.

- What it takes to comfort him—back patting or singing? shushing or rubbing his head?

As the coaching progresses, check the log daily and look for the following:

- Is your baby going to sleep quicker at the onset of sleep?
  - Is he waking fewer times at night?

- Is he staying awake at night for increasingly shorter periods of time?

- When he doesn't nap well, does he sleep poorly or get up too early the following night and morning?
  - Have there been any changes in his eating or health?

50

You can begin sleep coaching for naps when your healthy, full-term baby is six months old.

If your baby is healthy, growing well and is six months old, his day sleep should be organized and you can begin sleep coaching for naps. Remember that babies this age are rarely awake for more than three hours at a time, and they need two to three naps every day that are 45 minutes or longer. All told, that's three to three and a half hours of daytime sleep.

51

Early birds may get the worm—but it's no fun when they start chirping before 6 a.m.

If your baby gets up before 6 a.m., one of the following may be to blame:

- She's getting to bed too late. That's right—when you miss your baby's natural bedtime, she's more likely to wake frequently during the night and too early in the morning!

- She's too drowsy when she goes down at bedtime, so she hasn't yet mastered the art of putting herself to sleep. Then when she wakes at 5 a.m., after a nice long rest, she's going to have a really tough time getting back to sleep for another hour or so.

- She's nap-deprived and/or going too long between her afternoon nap and bedtime. This means she's heading to bed already sleep-deprived—with the stimulating hormone cortisol keeping her wired. In that condition, she's more likely to wake up early—and even more overtired.

52

Consistency is the key to sleep coaching — and parenting in general!

It's difficult to be consistent at two in the morning, when the easiest thing would be just to nurse a wakeful baby or bring him into bed. But being inconsistent (behavioral scientists call it "intermittent reinforcement") sends a mixed message. This makes sleep coaching more difficult for everyone!

There are three important ways in which you must be consistent:

• Respond to all of your child's wakings during the night the *same* way.

• Don't train your baby to cry. For example, if you stay to soothe your baby while he cries on and off, and after 15 minutes give up and rock or nurse him to sleep, you risk teaching him that if he just keeps crying, eventually you will do his bidding.

• Don't try to co-sleep part of the night and not others. Your baby can't tell time. Decide where you want your baby to sleep *all* night and then follow through with that plan until wake up time in the morning.

Children actually crave consistency. It reassures them to know what to expect and it helps them feel safe. It is truly the key to parenting, and especially to sleep success.

ABOUT KIM WEST

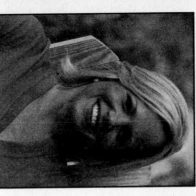

KIM WEST, the mother of two daughters, has been a practicing child and family social worker for more than fifteen years. Known as the Sleep Lady® by her clients, she has personally helped thousands of tired parents learn to listen to their intuition, recognize their baby's important cues and behaviors, and create changes that promote and preserve their child's healthy sleep habits.

Kim has appeared on *Dr. Phil*, *Today*, *NBC Nightly News*, *Good Morning America*, TLC's *Bringing Home Baby* and *CNN*, and has been written about in the *Wall Street Journal*, *Associated Press*, *Child* magazine, *Baby Talk*, *Parenting*, the *Baltimore Sun*, *USA Today* and the *Washington Post*, among other publications. West also hosts the sleep section of *The Newborn Channel*, which plays in maternity wards in hospitals across the country, and gives talks to parenting groups about the importance of children's sleep.

Kim is the author, with Joanne Kenen, of *GOOD NIGHT, SLEEP TIGHT: The Sleep Lady's Gentle Guide to Helping Your Child Go to Sleep, Stay Asleep and Wake Up Happy.* Published by Vanguard Press in January 2005, over 100,000 copies have been sold nationwide.

Kim West received her master's degree in Clinical Social Work from Simmons College in Boston and is a Licensed Certified Social Worker-Clinical (LCSW-C). She lives with her family in Annapolis, Maryland.

Visit Kim's website at *www.sleeplady.com* for more information and sleep resources, or to sign up for Kim's email newsletter.

BOOKS

GENERAL BABY AND CHILD CARE

Schmitt, Barton D., MD. *Your Child's Health: The Parent's One-Stop Reference Guide to Symptoms, Emergencies, Common Illnesses, Behavior Problems, and Healthy Development.* Bantam, 2005.

Shelov, Steven P., MD, FAAP. *Caring for Your Baby and Young Child: Birth to Age 5.* American Academy of Pediatrics, Bantam Doubleday Dell, 1998.

BEDTIME

Bauer, Marion Dane. *Sleep, Little One, Sleep.* Simon & Schuster, 2002.

Bentley, Dawn. *Good Night, Sweet Butterflies.* Simon & Schuster, 2003.

Boynton, Sandra. *Snoozers: 7 Short Short Stories for Lively Little Kids.* Little Simon, 1997.

Brown, Margaret Wise. *A Child's Good Night Book.* HarperCollins, 2000.

―――. *Goodnight Moon.* HarperFestival, 1991.

Dillard, Sarah (illustrator). *Ten Wishing Stars: A Countdown to Bedtime Book.* Intervisual Press, 2003.

Soft-to-Touch Books, *Good Night, Baby!* DK Publishing, 1995.

Fox, Mem. *Time for Bed.* Red Wagon Books, 1997.

Hague, Kathleen. *Good Night, Fairies.* Seastar Books, 2002.

Inkpen, Mick. *It's Bedtime, Wibbly Pig.* Viking, 2004.

Lewis, Kim. *Good Night, Harry.* Candlewick Press, 2004.

McBratney, Sam. *Guess How Much I Love You.* Candlewick Press, 1996.

McCue, Lisa. *Snuggle Bunnies*. Reader's Digest, 2003.

McMullen, Nigel. *It's Too Soon!* Simon & Schuster, 2004.

Meyer, Mercer. *Just Go to Bed*. Golden Books, 2001.

Munsch, Robert. *Love You Forever*. Firefly Books, 1986.

Paul, Ann Whitford. *Little Monkey Says Good Night*. Farrar, Straus and Giroux, 2003.

Rathmann, Peggy. *Good Night, Gorilla*. G. P. Putnam's Sons, 2000.

———. *10 Minutes Till Bedtime*. G. P. Putnam's Sons, 2001.

Steinbrenner, Jessica. *My Sleepy Room*. Handprint Books, 2004.

Trapani, Iza. *Twinkle, Twinkle, Little Star*. Charlesbridge Publishing, 1998.

BREASTFEEDING

Eiger, Marvin, MD, and Sally Wendkos Olds. *The Complete Book of Breastfeeding*. Workman Publishing, 1999.

Huggins, Kathleen, RN. *The Nursing Mother's Companion*. Revised edition. Harvard Common Press, 2005.

The Womanly Art of Breastfeeding. La Leche League International, 1997.

NEW SIBLING

Ballard, Robin. *I Used to Be the Baby*. Greenwillow, 2002.

Bourgeois, Paulette, and Brenda Clark. *Franklin's Baby Sister*. Scholastic, 2000.

Brown, Marc. *Arthur's Baby*. Little, Brown, 1990.

Henkes, Kevin. *Julius, the Baby of the World*. HarperTrophy, 1995.

London, Jonathan. *Froggy's Baby Sister*. Viking, 2003.

Meyer, Mercer. *The New Baby*. Golden Books, 2001.

MUSIC FOR RELAXATION AND BEDTIME ROUTINE

Ackerman, William. *The Opening of Doors.* 1992, Windham Hill Records

Baby's First Lullabies. 2005, Twin Sisters.

Disney Baby Lullaby: Favorite Sleepytime Songs for Baby and You. 1992, Walt Disney Records

Falkner, Jason. *Bedtime with the Beatles: Instrumental Versions of Classic Beatles Songs.* 2001, Sony Wonder.

Golden Slumbers: A Father's Lullaby. 2005, Rendezvous

Malia, Tina. *Lullaby Favorites: Music for Little People.* 1997, Music for Little People.

Music for Babies- Sleepy Baby. 2002, Big Kids Productions

Parents: The Lullaby Album. 1993, Angel Records.

Solnik, Tanja. *From Generation to Generation: A Legacy of Lullabies.* In Yiddish, Ladino, and Hebrew. 1993 and *Lullabies and Love Songs,* 1996, Dreamsong Recordings.

Stroman, Paige. *Lullabies to Celebrate Mother and Child.* 2001, National Music Marketing/Lullabyland.

WEBSITES

National Sleep Foundation
www.sleepfoundation.org
This nonprofit group addresses numerous sleep issues for children and adults. The website includes the group's new childhood sleep guidelines.

American Academy of Sleep Medicine (formerly the American Sleep Disorders Association)
www.aasmnet.org
The website of this membership group of doctors and other professionals contains links to sleep resources and research and also directs patients to accredited sleep disorder centers (not all of which treat children). Click "Patient Resources" to see a list of sleep disorder clinics.

American Academy of Pediatrics
www.AAP.org
The official site with advice and information about a multitude of pediatric topics. Resources, books and videos are available on their site.

Consumer Product Safety Commission
www.cpsc.gov
List of product recalls, safety requirements for various products such as cribs.

INFORMATION ON POSTPARTUM DEPRESSION

Medical Education on Postpartum Depression
www.MedEdPPD.org
An education website developed with the support of the National Institute of Mental Health. Updated information and resources for care providers and women with PPD.

Postpartum Support International
www.postpartum.net
Nationwide Helpline 1-800-944 4PPD (4773)
Provides current information, resources and education. Volunteer coordinators in every U.S. state and 26 countries who offer local support groups.

PHOTOS *(in order of appearance)*

Jack, *2 weeks old (cover)*

Philip, *6 months old*

Caden, *3 weeks old*

Adam, *2 months old*

Prairie, *1 month old*

Joshua, *7 weeks old*

Brady, *6 months old*

Lincoln, *almost 2 years old*

Nicholas, *11 months old*

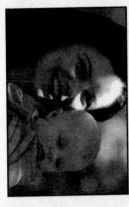

Dr. Lisa Thebner is a pediatrician in private practice in New York City. Dr. Thebner completed her residency training in Pediatrics at the Children's Hospital at Montefiore in the Bronx, New York, and graduated from the State University of New York at Buffalo School of Medicine and Biomedical Sciences. She is a Clinical Instructor in Pediatrics at New York Presbyterian-Weill Cornell Medical Center and is a regular medical contributor for Today in New York, the local WNBC news broadcast for the New York Metropolitan area. Dr.Thebner lives and sleeps through the night in New York with her husband, Eric Legome and baby daughter, Giselle.